A Year in the Life of a Medical Student Abroad

A Year in the Life of a Medical Student Abroad

Dr Costanza McIntosh

First published in the United Kingdom in 2020.

Self-published.

Copyright © Dr Costanza McIntosh 2020

The right of Dr Costanza McIntosh to be identified as the Author of the Work has been asserted by her in accordance with the Copyright, Designs and Patents Act 2020.

All rights reserved. No part of this publication may be reproduced, stored in a retrieval system, or transmitted, in any form or by any means without the prior written permission of the publisher, nor be otherwise circulated in any form of binding or cover other than in which it is published and without a similar condition being imposed on the subsequent purchaser.

Names, identities and circumstances have been changed in order to protect the privacy of the individuals involved. Please be aware that the information is not to be used in the diagnosis, treatment and prevention of disease and so all individuals must consult a medical professional for advice.

ISBN 9798571780292

This book is dedicated to my family because without their words of encouragement, support and prayers it would be impossible to be where I am today.

I am blessed.

Jeremiah 29:11

For I know the thoughts that I think toward you, saith the LORD, thoughts of peace, and not of evil, to give you an expected end.

Proverbs 16:3

Commit thy works unto the LORD, and thy thoughts shall be established.

God has a plan for every single one of us. This is your moment so why don't you claim it?

"My alma mater was books, a good library… I could spend the rest of my life reading, just satisfying my curiosity."

Malcolm X

Let's hope this book makes you feel just the same.

Fingers crossed…

Abbreviations

ALT: Alanine aminotransferase (enzyme to assist in determining liver function)
ASAP: As soon as possible
AST: Aspartate aminotransferase (enzyme to assist in determining liver function)
BP: Blood pressure
BTW: By the way
DDx: Differential diagnosis
Dx: Diagnosis
LDH: Lactate dehydrogenase
LOL: Laugh out loud
NEGL: Not even gonna lie
OCD: Obsessive compulsive disorder
PHx: Patient history
SMH: Shaking my head
TBH: To be honest

Preface

I must admit that I am a massive book worm. I have an insatiable appetite for reading and this is especially for books written by doctors talking about their lives and the patients that have made an impact on them and the way they practise. And what I love even more is when I find books written by doctors who specialise in my dream specialty-Infectious diseases/Tropical medicine. (Yes that's right show me a worm, talk about viruses or present to me a bacteria and I'll be a complete geek about it and won't even regret it LOL).

Throughout the years, I have found myself searching all over the internet for books written by medics studying away from their home countries. But this was with little success and so an idea popped into my head. DUH! Why not me?!

Studying abroad was one of the scariest yet amazing decisions I have made and it's truly unbelievable to see how far I have come. I have successfully completed my BSc in Biomedical Science in my home town of London, gone onto complete my Doctor of Medicine in Bulgaria and have now registered with the General Medical Council with a licence to practise. Won't God do it?!

On the other hand, I am sure that you may be wondering why on earth I am publishing my journal so late in my course. Well then I guess it's time to spill the beans.

It was literally just laziness really LOL. When I was younger I was never one to journal or keep a diary for more then a couple days due to boredom but now I am so glad I finally grew to enjoy it because it's quite nostalgic to have a means to look back and see whence you came from.

Admittedly, it's a shame I only started writing my journal in my fifth year of medical school however, it turned out to be my favourite year so I guess it worked out for the best in the end.

If you're wondering who this book is aimed at...

This book is for the 17 or 18 year old filling out their medical school application.

For the student rejected once again and wondering if their dreams of studying their favourite course at university will ever happen.

For the student who finds themselves in a school or country where most people don't look like them.

And for someone who just wants an honest and entertaining read whilst enjoying their cuppa before bed.

This is a book for every one-the medic and the non-medic alike.

So grab a snack.
Have a couple laughs.
Get cosy (and nosy LOL).
Be encouraged.
And hopefully learn something new.

Introduction

To me a life in the medical field is like no other. A solitary entity grounded on hard work, riddled with great sacrifice and yet is so raw in it's beauty that it is such a privilege to be apart of.

The highs and lows of life.
The frailty of humanity.
The magnitude of resilence.
The joy of recovery.
The warmth of compassion.

I am privileged to have the opportunity to be apart of it.

So now it's time for you to spend some time in my shoes.

Just for moment…

10th February 2019

Before I get into this book I would like to explain the first day I begun writing in my journal. It is funny how this decision came into existence almost at the end of my medical degree but oh well! Better late than never I'll say!

This journal was bought when I went on my first trip to Istanbul in November 2018. That is where I made a promise to myself to use it for something special. So, if I worked it out it would mean that this journal has literally been gathering dust on my shelf for at least three whole months.

Thankfully I inherited quality cleaning abilities from my Mum so maybe gathering dust is just an exaggeration LOL.

I also had to get my winter exams out the way first but thankfully they went well. Medical school exams are well known to be brutal but being in Bulgaria can push the limit that much more. The majority of our exams have a three step process of elimination as if you are being put through the Hunger Games (or so it feels like).

The first part is a selection of randomly allocated multiple choice questions and those who get the minimum pass mark can then proceed to the second stage. The second part involves writing a randomly chosen essay from the syllabus so everyone has to do their best to be equally competent in every topic as at least one (or even up to three) can be chosen. This can be so strenuous to prepare for especially as most modules have around 100 plus syllabus points. And then if you are successful you proceed to the third part which involves an oral exam with a doctor in that specialty lasting however long they choose. You better be prepared because they can talk about anything they want so it's best not to get the headshake of disapproval or you might get into a pickle I tell you that for sure.

An additional stage can be a practical involving you taking a history and doing a physical examination on a patient but that tends to be near the beginning (if that module has one included).

And for the majority of exams be prepared for a long day too! I have had exams that have started at 7:30am and not finished until after 6pm so describing them as long days is probably an understatement.

Some of the most difficult modules are the ones where there are multiple specialties being covered in one sitting such as our first internal medicine exam which included cardiology, pulmonology and TB medicine. What a day that was!

No matter how many times the examiners have read out the faculty numbers and/or names of those who have failed in front of the entire student body, it still feels nerve-racking every single time. And this can literally make your heart fall out your chest when some people have similar names to you. It's not fun but you do feel a massive sense of relief once it's all over and you have your red book in hand showing that you have passed. Freedom personified!

Anyways, the decision to write this journal was evoked by a very interesting and intellectually stimulating day at uni…

> **Winter exams results:**
>
> 07/01/2019
>
> Dermatology
> Passed with flying colours
>
> 14/01/2019
>
> Physiotherapy
> Passed with flying colours
>
> 21/01/2019
>
> Clinical Pharmacology
> Passed with flying colours
>
> 29/01/2019
>
> Anaesthesiology
> Passed (just about)
>
> 30/01/2019
>
> Orthopaedics & Traumatology
> Passed with flying colours

Fast forward...

21st February 2019

I dragged myself out of my bed for my 8am endocrinology practical but it was surprisingly well worth it. After completing a mini-test to review previous topics we covered, our teacher introduced us to two patients on the ward.

One of the patients was a middle aged male who had suffered chronic diarrhoea for a year. Now anyone who's had a stomach bug can attest to how gruesome constant rushes to the toilet can be due to the fact that you decided to eat leftovers from four nights ago out of laziness. (If this is you please DON'T. #studentproblems).

Unfortunately it was brought to our attention that this was related to his previous diagnosis of a pancreatic adenoma. (A pancreas is an abdominal organ in you body located posterior to the stomach which releases a lot of enzymes for digestion as well as hormones for regulation of your body's processes. Problems with it include issues with the hormone insulin which can lead to Diabetes Type 1 or 2 which I'm sure you've heard about at least once).

Our patient developed Diabetes Type 1 and so was put on a variety of medications including insulin (to replace the role of the pancreas in regulating glucose) as well as probiotics and Imodium (Loperamide) for his diarrhoea. (For some reason every time I hear or see the word Imodium I always recall that scene in the Big Bang Theory where Sheldon had to go to traffic court and the judge said "The court would advise you to make it quick, as the court had a dicey-looking breakfast burrito this morning and just took an Imodium."

(Side note: I am a Big Bang Theory fan and despite the show ending ages ago I still find myself watching old episodes and laughing at their jokes as if it was the first time).

But anyways, I digress.

With regards to the second patient who had given birth to a healthy boy a few months prior, her chief complaint was amenorrhea (missing menstrual periods). Some of my sister's friends call it "reds" but my friends and I prefer to call it our "time" whereas others prefer the better suited "worst days of the month" LOL.

(If you know, you know).

Bloods and MRI results confirmed that the cause was a ~12cm tumour in the pituitary gland (pea-sized gland in your brain that controls several other glands in the body). It was pretty massive so it was a surprise to us that she had no history of complaints before this admission when you consider its size and position.

However, after speaking to her further she brought up a key symptom which she had not raised before-she has been having a headache regularly for 10 years but thought that it was nothing to worry about and so didn't tell her GP about it.

Thankfully she has responded well to Bromocriptine (a dopamine agonist used to reduce the hormone prolactin which is being produced in excess due to the tumour) and because of this has regained her regular periods again.

After a break, it was time for Paediatrics. Knowing myself well, I know that I could not manage this specialty long term because I find it too emotional. I can see how it could get the brain juices flowing and it must be exciting seeing joyous kids with unparalleled resistance because they tend to bounce back very quickly but one must note that they can deteriorate equally as quickly.

We were not able to see paediatric patients presenting with the topic of that day so instead we found ourselves in an INTENSE session covering myocarditis and pericarditis (infections of the heart) with the professor.

The last session of the day was Forensic Pathology.

(Side note: If you enjoy such things like this I'd advise you to watch a programme called Dr G: Medical Examiner. Awesome show btw and you will learn an awful lot! My sister and I used to watch this show religiously on the weekends so take our word for it).

During the Forensic Pathology lesson we were able to go to the mortuary and see the examination of a suspected drowning. That was the first time I have seen a deceased body live in front of me. I must say that this is not for the fainthearted especially if this is not your sort of thing. But maybe I am a weirdo because I actually found it enthralling seeing our theoretical knowledge come to life "through death". Quite ironic really.

Tips I learnt from the Forensic Pathology session:

-Check the body for scars (they could be due to trauma or surgery for example)

-After a drowning, lungs become heavy and oedematous (fluid-filled)

-Always start from the head to the feet in order to be thorough with your examination

-Search for a possible causes e.g. strokes can lead to drowning

Three things I learnt today:

1. A common late sign of pancreatic adenomas is Type 1 Diabetes

2. Drowned victims typically have oedematous lungs and blood-tinged froth in their airways

3. Imodium and large burritos are a bad combo unless you want to stay glued to the toilet for 3 days

22nd February 2019

Currently barely keeping my eyes open.
It is still winter here so it's extremely dark outside. Understandable when it's 6:45am right now. Go figure.

Time to get ready for my first lesson of the day.

But the question is what should I wear?

Weather forcast?

3 degrees Celsius at this moment. Great (!)

Space suit it is…

Eventually I decided on a pencil skirt, top and thick coat. They say fashion is pain and my Mum always says "dress smart, think smart" so no other choice really.

Oh my!
I could not be happier!!!

Why you ask?

Well today I had my first Parasitology practical! (Such a geek-ish thing for me to say, I know right?) I have been waiting for this module for an eternity to tell you the truth.

During our lesson the teacher focused on the topic of that day- Diagnostic techniques but they also let us know that they just had a patient come into the clinic with Leishmaniasis who she would allow us to see after the lesson if we so desired.

This disease is caused by small parasites called trypanosomes and transmitted when sandflies bite. In this case, the area in which the patient stayed had many dogs which can be reservoirs of this parasite.

When she told us this it was nearly lunchtime so understandably the rest of the group wanted to grab something to eat before our next session whilst I stayed behind as an "eager beaver" to check out this patient.

To be fair it wasn't compulsory so the only reason I stayed behind was because it was related to my field of interest otherwise I'd be half through a portion of McDonald's fries at the mall by now.

Very interesting case.

Middle aged male
Visited Spain recently
Months of fever
Antibiotics proven ineffective
Pancytopenia (low platelet, erythrocyte and leukocyte count)
Hepatosplenomegaly (enlarged liver + spleen)
Positive serology

> *Classic presentation of Leishmaniasis = History of travel to endemic areas + fever + spleen involvement + pancytopenia*

The patient was placed on allopurinol (kills 1/10 parasites) and glucantime (This is a cardiotoxic drug so it is very important that ECGs are performed so that the patient's heart can be monitored properly). Glucantime was started at a dose of 20mg/kg and gradually increased to reduce the risk of toxicity.

23rd February 2019

WHY IS IT SNOWING?!!!

It has hardly snowed all winter and just as we are nearing spring the temperature plummets and I'm forced to wrap up and wear boots again.

(Hate boots btw).

Because the university campus is close to my apartment I decided to trudge through the snow and walk there. As I was making my way, I bumped into some students in my year group who had already been to the lecture room. Turns out that the lecture was CANCELLED! Just lovely (!) ☹

Back to bed then…

26th February 2019

2 questions.

Where on earth has the time gone?

Please can someone explain to me how we have practically reached the end of February already?

I only just celebrated New Years with the expectation that I had the whole year ahead of me but look how far we have reached already.

I guess it is a good time to buy Christmas presents whilst the deals are on!

*wink wink

I am absolutely exhausted but very happy the snow has melted. Don't get me wrong because as an avid photographer I love taking photos of the beauty that arises on a snow day BUT squelching through 10 inches of snow at 7am with fingers burning with frost doesn't exactly put a spring in your step, does it?

8am session.

The teacher was called in for an emergency surgery so they were unable to start until after 9am. Would have loved an extra hour sleep NEGL.

But I guess that is the unpredictability of medicine for you.

Thankfully the early start was worth it (again).

I was able to be present at my first C-section at 32 weeks gestation because the patient had developed severe preeclampsia (pregnancy complication where the mother experiences high blood pressure).

Good news! The baby should be fine after spending a few weeks in the neonatal department where their organs can get the time to develop and the mother is recovering well too.

> *When you are asked by an obstetrician where you are from but when you answer with the word "London" they feel that that cannot be. Apparently I can't be born and raised in the UK. Hmm. Microaggresions much! SMH*
>
> *Anyway we move...*

Endocrinology lecture.

The topic of today was thyroid disease so as a previous Graves' disease patient I found this one close to home. Graves' disease is an autoimmune condition where your immune system mistakenly attacks your thyroid which causes it to become overactive (hyperthyroidism) leading to symptoms such as anxiety, palpitations, extreme weight loss, sensitivity to heat and tremors. I was a textbook patient who if it wasn't for my Mum a nurse pleading with the GP to get me referred as a matter of urgency; I probably would not be here today.

Maybe I should write a book about it. Next book idea perhaps?

> *Although it was years ago, I am thanking God for my complete recovery. Health is fleeting so do not take it for granted.*

Psychology lecture.

To be completely honest, I was so baffled. The topic today was Nosology (classification) of Psychiatry.

Even so, I must say that he was one of the most enthusiastic lecturers I have ever had. He made the field come alive.

Massive kudos.

The plan for this evening:

- Get my workout out the way

- Prep my notes for tomorrow's lessons

    o   Murder my homemade cottage pie (I'm famished!)

Three things I learnt today:
1. Health is wealth

2. Every cause of hyperthyroidism is more common in women **except** for Toxic thyroid adenoma (benign thyroid tumour)

3. Always pack a snack because medical school will sap all your calories

I am hungry and knackered.
I think it will be an early night tonight.

27th February 2020

General medicine practical.

Was split into groups and assigned topics to research and talk about.

My group was given the topic cough which seems fairly simple but there's a lot to say. Moral of the story is coughs do not just occur because you have the flu. Coughs can arise from lung disease, heart disease and even after exposure to occupational hazards. One of these causes could be exposure to asbestos and funnily enough I know quite a bit about it. From when I was little my Dad has taught us about asbestosis. As an engineer it makes sense that he would find this fascinating but who would have thought that I would too!

Asbestos is a fibre often discovered in buildings for insulation but its use has been fully banned in the UK since 1999.

When patients come in with small particles of asbestos the damage is too far gone and because we do not currently have a cure the prognosis is poor. This fibre clings to lung tissue leading to irreversible inflammation and scarring.

Thankfully its use has reduced considerably however more must be done especially for resource-poor areas of the world (or what I like to call "countries-suffering-from-exploitation-and-colonial-rule," but that is a discussion for another day).

Psychiatry practical.

Today we discussed disturbances in emotion, memory, volition and consciousness. The best tip of the day was when the Professor told us that "laughter is necessary because without it we will not remember things."

I guess that's why even up to now I can still recall sentences from my favourite movies per verbatim but I struggle to remember the paediatrics notes I read yesterday evening. Maybe tears of exhaustion is not the best way to aid in memory but looking at the syllabus I know that there will be some tears of regret so let's see how that goes shall we?

Infectious Diseases lecture.

The lecturer discussed Rash syndromes.

Key infections to know in your practice regardless of specialty are chicken pox, scarlet fever, rubella and small pox.

Hopefully small pox doesn't rear its ugly head in the future but who knows? I am hoping that it doesn't but the UK voted for Brexit so anything is possible it seems.

Parasitology seminar.

Topic: Visceral and Cutaneous Leishmaniasis (Bye sandfly!)

General medicine lecture.

Topic: Family cycles of life.

I couldn't tell you what the lecturer was talking about because I conked out. I will definitely have to review this topic before the exam.

Three things I learnt today:

1. Laughter is not only the best medicine it's the best revision tool (apparently)

2. Leishmaniasis is caused by over 20 species of protozoa

3. The UK has officially lost it's marbles

28th February 2019

Endocrinology practical.

We saw a patient diagnosed with hypoparathyroidism and metabolic syndrome due to a prolactinoma (pituitary tumour overproducing prolactin) so the endocrinologist placed them on glucophage and destinox. The patient was referred to this department after they had visited their ophthalmologist complaining of a headache, fatigue as well as red bulging itchy eyes and so had been sent for a MRI scan which confirmed their suspicions.

Pediatrics practical.

Oh my gosh! I saw the cutest baby ever! They had large glistening eyes and were absolutely adorable. The poor thing had suspected RSV (Respiratory syncytial virus) that led to pneumonia and so had developed a stubborn cough and issues with breathing.

The mother did tell us that the older brother had come in a few days prior with the same infection so it is likely that they passed it to their sibling.

Forensic pathology lecture.

Topic: Different forms of asphyxia and post-mortem signs.

Oh no.
My tummy is so painful right now!

My lactose intolerance is acting up again. Being a cheese addict and having an intolerance of dairy is a vicious cycle that I hope one day I can break but I'm pretty confident that a plate of delicious, gooey Mac & cheese would send me back to my old ways so why pretend, eh?

(Side not: You're probably thinking I should try lactose-free cheese but to tell you the truth I absolutely detest it. Not my cup of tea at all mate LOL).

Three things I learnt today:

1.   No matter how you are feeling a cute baby will bring a massive smile to your face

2.   Signs of asphyxia

3.   Hypocalcaemia in very ill patients tends to mean the patient has a bad prognosis

1st March 2019

Pinch punch first day of the month!

Waking up to warmer temperatures really makes me happy.

18°C forecasted for this afternoon. #goals

8am- Paediatrics practical

Topic: Urinary tract infections (UTIs)

If you ever get a baby or infant with recurrent UTIs then it is probably a good idea to search for an anatomical cause. At this age, it could be a plethora of congenital abnormalities including vesicoureteral reflux (urine is pushed in the wrong direction due to problems with the valve) and horseshoe shape kidney (literally what it says on the tin).

Another of the babies admitted into the department had an IV line placed in their scalp which we found very odd. It was something I had not yet come across but it is used as an effective technique in various parts of the world but I had no idea. After speaking to the paediatrician and doing further research I came to find out that it is a stable and easy way to access their veins because in this region they do not have valves and that makes it a lot easier to advance the catheter when placing the IV line. Wow, you learn something new everyday!

Forensic pathology lecture.

Legit my favourite lecture of the week (I'm sure I've said this already). Not only is it an interesting specialty but we also have an exciting and well-read lecturer. You know the kind that inspires you to do more research or pick up that old textbook you've been avoiding.

Today's lecture they covered more forms of asphyxia including autoeroticism.

Wait a moment.

You're confused, right?

Don't worry you are not alone.

Because I was too.

This basically means people accidentally dying after attempting to reach sexual gratification using strangulation. I honestly didn't realise it was such a problem. In fact did you know that the USA has 500-1000 deaths due to this a year?

No?

Because I didn't.

What I love about this lecture is that the lecturer loves to get you learning actively so will randomly throw out a question to the audience.

I love this way of teaching. Quite fun actually.

Q: "Patient reports with neurological symptoms such as dizziness and ulcers on their fingers but only on the right hand."

Diagnosis?

Stunned silence. All of us found ourselves sifting through info in our brains trying to deduce the answer.

Then out of nowhere. A student (like a boss) raised their hand and with unmovable confidence said "Subclavian steal syndrome."

The rest of us waited with bated breath. Seconds felt like minutes…

The lecturer responds: "CORRECT!"

Again. Stunned silence.

They killed it!

> *Subclavian steal syndrome is cerebral ischaemia that results from diversion of blood flow from the basilar artery to the Subclavian artery due to occlusion. Because of this a new direction of blood flow is formed where it 'steals' blood from the opposite side.*
>
> *You probably will need to look into this further because I certainly had to. So I leave the extra research to you for tonight's homework.*

Three things I have learnt today:

1. Subclavian steal syndrome is a topic I need to read up on

2. Autoerotic asphyxia is a real issue

3. People will do anything to get that sexual "high"

Side note: Ratings to medical students in the US because those USMLE questions are no joke!

Bank holiday

Time for a lie in! I seriously felt like a cold is trying to get me.

Mum said I should get some cold meds as well as honey and lemon but let's see if I actually will.

(Spoiler alert: I didn't).

5th March 2019

Woke up with chills, fever and the feeling I had swallowed a frog whole so I skipped the first session-Obs & Gynae.

Forced myself to go in for my epidemiology practical where we discussed examples of vaccines and what happens pre- and post-exposure. Apparently my teacher says that Hep B recombinant vaccine is the safest so I will have to do my own research on why that is.

I only managed to attend one lecture as opposed to the three scheduled for today.

Thanks to the flu(!)

Endocrinology lecture.

Topic: Hyperparathyroidism and Hypoparathyroidism

Hypoparathyroidism is decreased function of the parathyroid glands whereas hyperparathyroidism is increased function of the parathyroid glands. Parathyroid glands are four small glands which regulate calcium levels in our bodies and are found in your neck.

During this lecture the teacher kept stressing to us how tired she was hearing students say that both types caused osteoporosis because it showed lack of knowledge. She made it emphatically clear that this makes no sense at all and after the rant was over ended with a chuckle.

Fingers crossed that I won't be one of them.

To my medics out there…

For the sake of peace and to avoid chastisement from your examiner you should probably remember this schematic diagram:

> *Hyperparathyroidism:*
>
> ↑*parathyroid hormone* → ***increased** activity of osteoclasts (bone cells that produces calcium by breaking down bone)* → *increased breakdown of bone (osteoporosis)*
>
> *Hypoparathyroidism:*
>
> ↓*parathyroid hormone* → ***decreased** activity of osteoclasts* → *bone remains intact*

Three things I have learnt today:

    1.   My immunity is as effective as a paper bag in the rain

    2.   I need to get my tetanus booster because it's overdue

    3.   Hypoparathyroidism DOES NOT lead to osteoporosis

Oh right. Time for bed now.

6th March 2019

Feeling a little better than yesterday. Maybe that multivitamins drink I got has helped? Who knows?

7:45am General medicine practical

Last week the teacher asked us to prep notes on various symptoms commonly encountered by GPs including nausea, vomiting, diarrhoea and chest pain. It was a very informative lesson.

This time around my group and I were assigned the topic nausea. It actually made me realise how much more complicated nausea was and the fact that it could be linked to so many diseases from the mundane like a self limiting viral stomach bug to the sign of something life threatening like head trauma or meningitis. The teacher seemed very content with what we said and so we were well chuffed. ☺

Here are some of my notes:

Nausea is the urge to vomit. The main sites of control of nausea are the vomiting centre (VC) in the medulla and the chemoreceptor trigger zone in the medulla. The medulla is one of the most if not the most important part of the brain and controls involuntary functions including breathing and heart rate. When you slice through it kind of looks like a cauliflower. (Not to put you off your food but I have confirmed this watching multiple autopsies btw so bear with me LOL).

Anyways.

There are multiple pathways that can lead to nausea and vomiting:

- Cortex: When we are anxious or have increased pressure in the head e.g. meningitis we can activate the VC

- Chemoreceptor trigger zone: When the brain picks up toxins in the blood or CSF e.g. alcohol (Most students know exactly what I'm talking about here #freshersweek. I don't drink myself but I've watched enough people that do and it's not for me periodt)

- Peripheral: Irritation of nerves particularly in the gastrointestinal tract e.g. after last night's dodgy takeaway

- Vestibular: Irritation of the vestibulocochlear nerve (for hearing and balance) by infection etc

> *Pop quiz time!*
>
> *What number cranial nerve is the vestibulocochlear nerve?*
>
> *Tick tock.*
>
> *I surely hope you remembered that it is number eight.*
>
> *You didn't?*
>
> *(Just kidding. I forgot myself. Thank God for Google! LOL)*

Effectively your role as GP (if you decide to pursue this profession) will be to decipher through the patient's history and find the trigger for the nausea.

Also don't forget to rule out the simplest causes that we often forget.

PREGNANCY FOR EXAMPLE!!!

It's not everyday you'll find yourself frantically searching through the National

Organization for Rare Disorders website. Most times the answer is right before you. #occamsrazor

After this practical I had a short break followed by our last practical of the day- Psychiatry.

Topics:
- Antipsychotics
- Antidepressants
- Mood stabilisers
- Tranquilizers

The professor took us to where they store the psych meds and went through commonly prescribed drugs. Some of it is a blur but it was fascinating from what I remember.

Ironically, it is not uncommon to find medical students depending on meds like these to try and get through learning all the information taught in university. After this intense session I can see the reasons why but please don't deal with this alone! It's not worth it. Never be too afraid to talk to someone and seek professional help ASAP.

We also met a middle aged woman with depression exacerbated by loneliness and the fact that her children had all left home. (Unfortunately this is a common occurrence so if you haven't already please check up on your parents and older relatives every so often because they probably won't say it but they'd appreciate it. After all one day that will be you).

> *Psalm 71:9 (KJV)*
> *Cast me not off in the time of old age;*
> *forsake me not when my strength faileth.*

Three things I have learnt:

1. Pharmaceutical companies are never really going to struggle for cash

2. The importance of spelling medications properly when prescribing especially when most doctors have TERRIBLE handwriting

3. Medicine is not easy but it is okay to let someone you trust know because from my experience a problem shared really is a problem halved

7th March 2019

No clue why but today the group was giddy with tiredness. We found ourselves making jokes and laughing throughout the lessons.

Diagnosis: MIDS

i.e. Medical Student Delirium Syndrome

Treatment: A good eight to nine hours of uninterrupted sleep

Prognosis: Poor (Because getting this many hours of sleep as a medical student is pretty much impossible)

Endocrinology practical.

Topic: Hyperparathyroidism (again)

We had a replacement endocrinology teacher today due to the fact that our normal teacher was unavailable. Sad to say this but it was actually one of the best endocrinology practicals I have had.

She was so clear and concise with her explanations and asked thought provoking questions and gave us scenarios to help cement what we had learnt.

Dear Dr A thanks for that.

I have no choice but to drop you some straight bars from the lesson:

Clinical features of hyperparathyroidism include:

- Epilus (mandibular/lower jaw tumours)

- Proximal muscle weakness (there are times where the muscles are so weak they can even pull away from the joints they are normally attached to)

- Diabetes inspidus (reduced sensitivity to antidiuretic hormone leading to weak urine)

- Peptic ulcers

- Pancreatitis

- Cholelithiasis (gall bladder stones)

- Depression

The most common cause of hyperparathyroidism is benign tumours in the parathyroid glands so often surgery is the best way forward.

And do you remember from a previous diary log that it can lead to osteoporosis?

I hope that's a yes!

With those with osteoporosis it is important to remember that patients often do not even realise that they have had a fracture and it is stumbled upon haphazardly on X-ray.

> Tip: For these patients aim for a Vitamin D level of approximately >30 nanograms per litre

Paediatrics practical:

The first patient was a teenage male with lower back pain that started a couple days ago:

• Swollen eyes in the morning (periorbital oedema)

• Microscopic hematuria (blood in the urine that is invisible to the naked eye)

• Elevated creatinine levels (indicates poor kidney function)

- BP: 140/200 (when the diastole or bottom number is elevated it is suggestive of hypertension due to something wrong with the kidneys)

> *Children are not mini adults in fact I remember hearing a surgeon say that adults were older children considering the way they act LOL.*
>
> *Here is a helpful tip to help you decide if a child has hypertension.*
>
> *Systole (top number) = 90 + 2X years*
> *Diastole (bottom number) = 60 + years*
>
> *This calculation gives a rough idea of what their blood pressure should be.*
>
> -----------
>
> *Tip 2: Renal oedema tends to be found in the face/ upper body and more apparent in the morning whereas cardiac oedema tends to be found on the lower limbs and more visible as the day progresses.*

Also, we saw an eight year old boy with a rash, swollen hands, abdominal pain and a BP of 120/70. (I will leave it to you to work out if this is normal or not for his age).

Diagnosis: Henoch-Schönlein purpura (inflammation of the blood vessels leading them to become leaky and so a rash forms most often on the lower body).

The doctor has put the cause down to a previous bout of tonsillitis because Henoch-Schönlein purpura is often triggered by infection or allergy. *I definitely keep spelling this incorrectly so I had to double check when writing this.*

That's why having an in depth history and examination should form the bulk of your decision making. Be thorough. Listen carefully. And eventually the patient's body will tell you the answer.

Forensic practical.

We discussed the findings for asphyxia for autopsies.

Carotid compression can lead to arrhythmia whereas compression of the jugular vein tends to lead to brain oedema.

There are multiple types of asphyxia including:

- Neck compression
- Chest compression
- Airway obstruction
- Exhaustion of oxygen

Is it weird to be excited about seeing an autopsy?

Because apparently there is a possibility that one may be happening tomorrow morning and I am intrigued.

Medics really have issues don't we? LOL

Also I am looking forward to my parasitology practical tomorrow too (obviously)!

Three things I have learnt today:

1. Washerwoman skin is a term used in Forensics for when the skin of the body appears dry and wrinkled after being immersed in water for a prolonged period of time

2. Medics are complete weirdoes

3. I need to work on my spelling pronto

8th March 2019

Currently I am chilling in my bed watching mukbangs on Youtube, as you do. Clearly I have an unhealthy relationship with food that borders on the level of OCD. I'm a food enthusiast and that also includes watching others eating and talking about food.

Admittedly I'm weird but for one.

Who isn't?

And two.

If you have read this far than you really shouldn't be surprised.

Also I had my favourite lecture and my favourite practical today so I am well haps!

Parasitology practical.

Got to meet the patient with Leishmaniasis again to see how he was getting on since I last saw him (this time the whole class was there too). I learnt some new things about the case so medicine is the gift that just keeps giving it seems.

His haemoglobin was low but this is expected to get to normal levels after completion of treatment. The teacher also showed us how ampoules of glucantime actually looked and once again stressed to us how toxic it is.

Apparently if this drug was bought in the US it would cost 20,000 USD. Unbelievable! Thankfully here in Bulgaria it only costs about 300 Euros.

Miltefosine may also be helpful and is an anticancer dug as well. I also vaguely remember it being used with other drugs for termination of pregnancies but don't quote me on this.

I don't think it's the time to get political because if I start I will never finish but if you want to know my views we might have to write another book in the future.

> **Evidently I've completely mixed up two drugs but we move...**
>
> *Miltefosine* vs *Mifepristone*

Rooky mistake. This is why you can find junior doctors scrolling through the BNF app on wards in the UK to reduce mishaps like this.

Eek. My bad.

Anyways...

DRUGS USED FOR THE TERMINATION OF PREGNANCY:

Mifepristone *is taken orally. This drug counters the effect of progesterone, a hormone necessary for pregnancy.*

Misoprostol *is almost always used in conjunction with mifepristone to induce a medical abortion. Misoprostol is a prostaglandin-like drug that causes the uterus to contract.*

Methotrexate *is used less often but may be used in women who are allergic to mifepristone.*

Oh my gosh! We got the chance to see Leishmania parasites under the microscope. So cool!

We also discussed other infections such as Entamoeba histolytica infection, Cryptosporidiosis and Giardiasis.

I didn't make these words up btw.

But what is the connection between them?

Pause.

Got the answer?

Well, they tend to be due to contaminated food or water and can lead to intestinal infection.

That's why you can't eat from everyone you know.

(Bless your food whilst you're at it guys.)

Forensic Pathology lecture.

Topic: Blunt force trauma.

Very informative but I expected nothing less from this lecturer.

As always he ended the lecture with scenario questions to test our knowledge but this time from the MRCP part 1 in Neurology. *MRCP is an abbreviation for Member of the Royal College of Physicians and is used to examine doctors who hope to specialise in their chosen field like neurology for example.*

Way beyond our pay grade but it was fun attempting.

Some helpful algorithms I gathered from the questions:

> *Risk of thrombosis + bumping into things (despite no visual complaints) =*
>
> *Anton's syndrome*

This disease is fascinating because the brain literally makes up what the patient sees to compensate for vision loss. How mind-boggling.

> *Upper lower neuron signs + lower motor neuron signs + normal sensation = Amyotrophic lateral sclerosis*
>
> --------
>
> *Reduced immunity/elderly patient + meningitis symptoms = Listeria monocytogenes*
>
> -------
>
> *High temperature + seizures + temporal lesion = HSV encephalitis*

The lecturer said that you can diagnose over 100 diseases just by looking at the nails of your patient. Who would have thunk it?

9th March 2019

Hate Saturday lectures-they are really the banes of my existence.

And so because of this I cannot really say what on earth the lecturer was banging on about today but managed to catch some Zzs. LOL

Clinical oncology lecture.

Blah blah blah. (Drifting in and out of sleep).

Well at least it's a sunny day today!

Sometimes you really need that Vitamin D kick so I found myself walking with a spring in my step on my way home but to tell you the truth this might just be me rejoicing that the lecture was finally over.

On another note I have reached home now. Finally. (The perks of living close to your university campus).

Now I am doing the usual. Catching up on YT subscriptions and ended up stumbling across a video about university applications and rejection.

Ironically if anyone could relate to this it would definitely be me because I too have gone through my own share of rejections.

1) 2001- Went through the whole rigmarole of UCAS in choosing and applying to four medical schools and one backup (I mean, who thought of that? It really makes sense to reduce the options from 5 to 4 for an already competitive course, right? Illogical in my opinion but I doubt that'll change). Honestly I cannot even remember the universities I applied for but what I do know is that they all said a big fat NO.

To be fair my UKCAT grade was a joke so it does make sense now I think about it. I have my own views on that "aptitude test" however once again that is a discussion for another day.

2) 2014- Nearing the end of my BSc in Biomedical Science and once again did the whole UCAS gobbly gook. And you guessed it, got a NO from every university I applied to. Graduate medicine is known to be even more competitive than undergraduate medicine and I don't think

an average score at UKCAT (for the second time) helped either.

But then...

A silver lining...

3) Applied to medical school in Bulgaria in spring 2014 and a few months later in summer 2014 as I made my way home from university I received an email notification from the agency sorting out my application. Clicked on it and saw the words "You have been successful..."

(Unfortunately that company has dissolved now but I am thankful they existed to help make this opportunity possible).

Pure jubilance! I was bursting with excitement and couldn't wait to get home to tell my parents the good news! Even today, when I think back to this moment I cannot help but smile.

Letting my grandparents know the good news a few days later face-to-face is another moment that I will never forget. Seeing my grandfather jump out of his seat, eyes bright with pride and joy is another moment that I have not forgotten even up to today. Sometimes in my darkest moments in medical school I would replay this moment in my mind for strength. For this, I am grateful that he was able to be apart of this process before God called him home to glory a few months before my medical school graduation. Without him I wouldn't be where I am today so I feel blessed for this.

    Rest easy Grandad.

What have these highs and lows taught me?

Rejections must be perceived as redirections because often what was initially seen as a disappointment turns out to be an appointment to something greater.

Diamonds are made under high pressure and heat and so situations such as these will either break you or make you. I choose to become stronger. I can truly attest to this, because looking back I have achieved more then I even anticipated but more importantly I have grown exponentially.

The 2011 Costanza is not the 2019 Costanza.

I have made great friends.

I have developed new skills.

I have had some amazing teachers who are inspirational physicians.

And in all of this my passion for medicine has grown and I am that much closer to what I was called to do.

So I say this to say to you that you should keep on pushing.

If it may be applying for medicine or trying to raise funds for that business venture or trying to find ways to help your community your time will come.

You must persevere, drown out the noise and distractions and keep focused on the goal. If you quit or throw in the towel the minutes, days and years will continue to pass so you might as well try, right?

I know it's such a random motivational speech but who knows maybe this diary entry was just as much for me as it was for you?

Well, I'm off to have a nap now.

(Boy am I predictable SMH).

11th March 2019

I only have one lesson today, thank God.

Endocrinology practical @ 9:30am.

We didn't see patients today but discussed Diabetes Type 1 & 2.

The teacher said that we will discuss medications next lesson so we should read up on them beforehand. Funnily enough that will be our last endocrinology lesson before we start the next rotation- gastroenterology.

Bye bye pituitary adenomas and diabetes and hello ulcers and cirrhosis.

I am looking forward to learning something new but endocrinology was fascinating so I hope gastroenterology will be too. Neither of them can even come close to Tropical medicine as a specialty but I guess it was a good try.

Later today I was supposed to be attending the Paediatrics lecture but to be brutally honest I do not find the lectures particularly helpful and so I prefer to go through the material on my own.

So home it is.

12th March 2019

Bunked the Obs & Gynae practical but hoping to not make this a habit.

Fingers crossed.

Infectious Diseases practical.

We were given a test to do on CNS infections and went through a couple of cases.

1) Teenage boy with meningitis due to the bacteria *Neisseria meningitidis*

2) Middle aged woman presenting with seizures and a temporal lobe lesion on CT due to HSV encephalitis (I hope you've remembered this one from a previous diary log on those MRCP questions I was talking about before, right? If not, I am disappointed LOL)

Funny how I just saw this previously during the Forensic Pathology lecture a few days ago and it has come back to haunt me.

> *Moral of the story: Medical school is about linking topics together so try your best to keep up to date with the material regularly*

Endocrinology lecture.

Topic: Diabetes Type 1 & 2

(Last endocrinology lecture of the year!)

Three things I have learnt today:

1) Females with polycystic ovarian syndrome (PCOS) are 5-7 times more likely to develop diabetes in their lifetime

2) Learn well because different specialties interconnect so you will probably encounter that particular disease again

3) If you suspect meningitis in a teenage/adult patient always test for the bacteria *Haemophilus influenzae*, *Streptococcus pneumoniae* and *Neisseria meningitidis* as they are the likely culprits

Just quickly jotting this down before I do my workout. Probably not said this before but I started to try to incorporate more exercise into my week about 2 years ago.

It began with walking around the park but that died a death pretty quickly. Then I thought of joining the gym and that never happened. Facepalm.

How then, you ask?

Home workouts are the way. I try to exercise about three or four times a week doing high intensity exercise for about 30 minutes max. Could do more but ain't nobody got time for that! LOL

I try to get mostly cardio in and focus on a specific body part on different days.

Today's actually abs/cardio day so wish me good luck!

Back to today's recap...

General medicine practical.

We had it in the simulation centre where we got to use the very life-like dolls in order to practice auscultation of the lungs to enable a more accurate differential diagnosis. It was quite fun actually. I thoroughly enjoyed the detective work today. And it makes it even better that we have an awesome teacher. #inspired

Psychiatry practical.

We discussed psychotic disorders and then saw a teenage patient recently diagnosed with schizophrenia.

Infectious Disease practical.

We learnt about a meningococcal disease caused by *Neisseria meningitidis*. The lecturer also brought up a syndrome that I've come across whilst researching when I was at secondary school called Waterhouse–Friderichsen syndrome. This is where the adrenal glands severely bleed and fail due to this infection. It is a very dangerous but fascinating complication of infection by this bacterium.

Parasitology lecture.

Absolutely hilarious session.

My lecturer is such an animated and cheeky character so he often keeps me awake even when I'm exhausted so well done Professor.

It also helps that I love the subject.

Some of the infections we looked at:
- Amoebiasis
- Acanthamebiasis
- Trichomonas vaginalis
- Toxoplasmosis
- Pneumocystisis

The lecturer also let us know that he's been to quite a few places for work and studied in Egypt. He also started asking if any of us know Spanish and ended up going of on a tangent with one of the Spanish students.

General medicine lecture.

Please don't ask me what on earth the lecturer was talking about mate?!

This is for three reasons:

- They had no microphone so we could barely hear them

- The lecturer was banging on about schemes (really should of tried to listen more intently but it is what it is)

- It was one of the driest lectures I've ever attended

You win some you lose some, I guess.

Three things I have learnt today:

1) Leucopoenia (low white blood cell count) can be a sign of severe bacterial infection

2) I need to get my tetanus booster…still

3) Getting distracted in boring lectures is dangerously easy

14th March 2019

The colder weather has returned. ☹

On my way to my lesson I decided to pop into the local shop and buy an aloe drink in the flavour peach for the first time. It was not bad at all. But this one had pulp so it may not be to everyone's liking.

Endocrinology practical @ 8am.

Last endo practical in this rotation.

We did a review test which surprisingly was do-able.

Saw three patients with diabetes and they were all on insulin.

The teacher discussed different types of antidiabetic meds. Because I love pharmacology I found it very interesting. But I must admit that when the teacher put two handfuls of insulin pens in front of us and asked us to group them based on their properties we found that quite tricky. I probably need to read up on them because evidently I know the oral medications e.g. metformin better than I know the different forms of insulin.

> *Insulin products can be divided by their duration of action from ultra-short acting to long acting.*
> *Tip: Given as a subcutaneous injection (below the skin)*

Paediatrics practical @10:15am.

Premature baby
Low birth weight
Jaundice
Increased LDH, bilirubin, AST & ALT (indicates liver disease)
Hepatomegaly (enlarged liver)

PHx: Heart murmur, anaemia
Dx: Neonatal hepatitis

She was so small that when you held her you felt like you could break her. I am hoping that she makes a speedy recovery. ☹

> *To remember possible causes of neonatal hepatitis use the mnemonic **TORCH**:*
>
> ***T**OXOPLASMOSIS*
> ***O**THER (e.g. syphilis)*
> ***R**UBELLA*
> ***C**MV*
> ***H**ERPES VIRUS*

Forensic Pathology practical.

We discussed wounds, abrasions and lacerations. It amazes me how forensic pathologists can determine the age of a wound just from a mere look.

After this we attended an autopsy of an elderly male killed in a road traffic accident. The injuries were absolutely horrific and so that was one that I will never forget. *I urge you to please drive safely guys!*

Three things I learnt today:

1. There's way more types of insulin than I thought

2. I can fit 2 large segments of oranges in my mouth (I actually figured this out after a dare my group forced me

into during our lunch break. We really are loonies. SMH)

3. Abrasions heal without scars whereas lacerations are irregular, have tissue bridges and heal with scars

15th March 2019

The weather forecast really fooled me today. It was predicted to be around 10°C but walking out I was confronted with intense sunshine so guess I didn't need my coat. Oh well. I can't complain to be fair. I'd take the heat over the cold any day. Also my mum has a habit of saying that it's better to have it and not need it then need it and not have it. So here we are.

I had a very unusual paediatrics patient today the young girl was complaining of vomiting, abdominal pain and diarrhoea. It turns out that she has Fanconi anaemia (congenital aplastic anaemia where they have a very low blood cell count). Patients with this disorder are infection prone and she needed a bone marrow transplant and so had to travel to another country to receive it a few months prior.

The teacher reminded us that the riskiest post-transplant period is up to 3 months following their transplant surgery. Engraftment (body accepts donor organ) starts around the 20th day after surgery and the patient has low platelets so they will be transfusion dependent for now. Because of this bone marrow dysfunction as well as the fact that they have been put on immunosuppressant medications to reduce the risk of rejection there is a very huge risk of infection which is the most likely reason for her admission today.

In transplant patients it is helpful to know that in the first months it makes sense to expect a fungal cause and after that suspect a viral cause of infection. In cases such as these, it is a must that those in the medical field are weary of a very dangerous virus Cytomegalovirus (CMV). Unfortunately this is exactly what our patient had so she had to be put on a long course of antiviral drugs including Ganciclovir and Acyclovir.

> *Make sure that if you are involved in a transplantation procedure that you know the signs of graft-versus-host-disease (GVHD) where the donor cells attack the recipient's cells.*

> *Early signs include erythema (redness) and bulla (blisters).*
>
> *Late signs are due to the deposition of antibodies and include hyperpigmentation (darkening of the skin) and gastrointestinal complaints such as vomiting and diarrhoea.*

Forensic Pathology lecture.

Topic: Abrasions, lacerations and brain injuries

I was excited to come in today and for good reason. The lecturer did his usual quizzing on different scenarios from the MRCP Neurology part 1 again. It was exciting to become a neurologist for a short moment.

Some interesting cases:

- Teen, dysarthria (issues with speech), tremors and psychosis

<u>Dx: Wilson's disease (genetic disease leading to a build up of copper)</u>

- Young patient with biphasic brain activity on EEG and memory loss six months ago

Dx: Creutzfeldt–Jakob disease (mad cow disease)

> Moral of the story:
> Avoid eating raw meat

Okay I'm done for the day now.
Time for a much needed (fully cooked) meal.

16th March 2019

I was so peckish so I had to come home to make something to eat before I even was able to update you guys about my day.

Saturday lectures are pure evil so when I heard my alarm this morning I thought someone was pranking me. One thing you should know about me (unless you've already figured out) is that I hate waking up early in the mornings. I am definitely not an early bird at all!

Clinical Oncology lecture.

Once again tapped out of the lecture within the first few minutes but I do vaguely remember something about the words "oncological emergencies," "tumour lysis syndrome," "hypercalcaemia" and "superior vena cava syndrome."

Setting you homework to research some terms once again.

18th March 2019

First day of the week. The time is now 7:46pm.

Just finished my workout and remembered that I haven't written anything today. Anyways we only had one lesson today (our second internal diseases rotation)- gastroenterology. This lesson didn't really last very long as it was just an introductory lesson. It involved us signing forms and getting a tour of the department. We also were given a test to see what we knew. And too be fair it was pretty easy so no worries at all.

19th March 2019

Random thought but I just woke up so bare with me.

Sound of birds chirping…

Is it only me that finds it so fascinating how the birds are able to wake up in sync with the sunrise? They're so in tune with nature it really makes you appreciate the beauty around us. With this in mind, I do wish I could wake up with such ease but unfortunately that's virtually impossible.

It's around 7:30am right now and even though my body is comfortable where it is I have no choice but to move because it's time to get ready for uni now (unfortunately).

Today's lessons should include an obs & gynae practical, epidemiology practical and then three lectures (gastroenterology, psychiatry and obs & gynae) but I'll probably only go to the practical and first lecture today instead.

I really cannot be asked to go to all of them today.

For the psych lecture I feel like I need my own evaluation because I always leave baffled by what on earth the lecturer is banging on about. And with regards to the Obs & Gynae lecture I find it much easier to grasp within the comfort of my home TBH. The younger me used to try and attend every lecture but if you are disciplined enough and know how to plan your time you can adjust your timetable accordingly especially when you know you'll only end up spending the next 2 hours in REM sleep as opposed to actually digesting what the lecturer presents.

On another note I'm so hungry. I hope this banana will suffice until I can have something proper to eat because this won't do. #potassiumhit

20th March 2019

General medicine practical.

Our time in the general medicine practical was spent in the medical simulation centre practising auscultation of heart murmurs with our teacher. It was a fun but helpful lesson. I definitely need more work but practice makes perfect so we will get there.

Psychiatry practical.

We have to go up a very steep hill in order to get to the psychiatry department.

Wow that was a workout!

Today we discussed depression and bipolar disorder and met an elderly woman with panic disorder. She was so lovely and even showed us some black & white photos of her and her husband at her wedding day.

The elderly can be so cute sometimes. Bless them.

Epidemiology lecture.

Topic: Hepatitis A, B, C & D

Did you know that Hepatitis B can remain stable outside of the body in dried blood for over a week? Yikes!

Parasitology lecture.

ESSENTIALLY LOTS OF WORMS

Our lecturer told us a story about his time in Vietnam where he performed an autopsy on a male with over a thousand worms in his intestine. Funny how some of these worms for example *Taenia saginata* (pork tapeworm) can grow to over 5 metres long! That's nearly as tall as me. Unbelievable!!! *Guess that'll put you right off your spaghetti. LOL.*

General medicine lecture.

Topic: The role of GPs in palliative care

To tell you the truth I don't find the lecturer particularly engaging and the aesthetic of the lecture slides doesn't help either. Different strokes for different folks, I guess.

Three things I learnt today:

1. The Hepatitis B virus is one tough cookie

2. Don't make spag bol for dinner on the day of your parasitology lecture

3. 25% of the world is infected by the same type of worms including *Ancylostoma duodenale*

21st March 2019

Gastroenterology practical.

This was the quickest practical ever and lasted only for 10-15 minutes discussing gastro-oesophageal reflux disease (GERD).

Paediatrics practical.

We discussed questions on nephrology and gastrointestinal issues in children.

Forensic Pathology practical.

This autopsy was one that will stick with me forever. A young person was found in his vehicle having died of a sudden cardiac arrest. On examination left ventricular hypertrophy (enlarged heart) and heart disease was found. Considering his age and the fact that he was only a year younger than me it really shook me up a bit. Moments like this makes you really appreciate life.

Enjoy life. Spend time with your loved ones because you never know.

Since I had a break, I decided to ask the Infectious Diseases doctor if I could shadow her later on today whilst she was on duty. She said yes, so in my excitement I decided to treat myself to a new chocolate bar from Lidl. It deserves a 10/10! No clue if this was because I was so peckish or because it was actually that good but I guess I will have to buy another one to confirm it. *I'm supposed to cut down on the snacks I eat but I have to do what is necessary in the interest of science, right?* *wink wink

Three things I learnt today:

1.   Haemolytic Urea Syndrome (HUS) = haemolytic anaemia (breakdown of red blood cells) + renal failure + thrombocytopenia (low platelet count)

2.   There are different types of nephrotic syndrome (kidneys leak a lot of protein into the urine) including selective proteinuria (only leaks small proteins that can pass through the membrane) and non-selective proteinuria (leaks small and large proteins)

3.   There are instances where giving milk to newborns is contraindicated such as when they have been diagnosed with liver disorders such as galactosemia (galactose in the blood) or tyrosinemia (tyrosine in the blood)

Shadowing the ID doctor.

I only spent about an hour with her whilst she was on duty.

Middle aged woman
Extreme headache
Fatigue
Memory loss
PHx: Had multiple operations on her nose for rhinorrhoea (discharge from the nose) and polyps
A brain malformation was found on MRI

She has been given mannitol (reduces the brain oedema), steroids (reduces inflammation), painkillers and antibiotics.

Also saw a young girl who came in with mood changes and ataxia (lack of control and coordination) due to cerebritis (inflammation of the brain) as a complication of chicken pox. Thankfully she is doing very well and will be discharged in a couple of days. ☺

22nd March 2019

Thank God it's Friday.

I have never been so excited to come home to bed!

Paediatrics practical.

Very interesting patient:

Infant male
Born premature and had suffered an intra-amniotic (inside the womb) infection
History of many infections since birth including:

- Bronchitis

- Cervical lymphadenitis (inflammation of lymph nodes in neck)

- Pneumonia

- Peritonsillar (around the tonsils) abscess

- Fungal Oesophagitis (inflammation of the oesophagus)

Their blood test showed low neutrophils and high eosinophils. Genetic testing was advised and a diagnosis was finally made.

Dx: Myeloid differentiation primary response 88 disorder

I have honestly never heard of this disorder at all in my life so if you're confused you're not the only one, trust me.

(Thank God once again for the internet).

This rare disorder is a defect in the Myeloid differentiation primary response 88 (MYD88) protein which orchestrates the signalling that occurs in your immune system and so these patients are very susceptible to bacterial and fungal infections.

> *This patient reminded me of a lesson I had during my first degree-Biomedical Science where we were told a tip "Remember the most common signs and symptoms for the rarest diseases and remember the rarest signs and symptoms for the most common diseases."*

Definitely relevant today!

Parasitology practical.

Malaria!!!

Even got to see some thin and thick smears under the microscope.

Apologies for geeking out but…

Yay!!! So cool ☺

Forensic Pathology lecture.

Topic: Injuries due to sharp objects.

Three things I learnt today:

1. You need at least 50 parasites per microlitre of blood to detect malaria using a microscope

2. *Plasmodium malariae* is a parasite that causes malaria and can lead to immune complex nephritis (inflammation of the kidneys due to the deposition of antibodies) in children

3. The antibiotic Doxycycline can cause a photosensitive rash (skin reaction to light) yet it is prescribed in countries that typically get a lot of sun (make it make sense please?)

23rd March 2019

Our teacher messaged one of the students in my group last night to let us know that today we could watch a full autopsy! It will be the first time I see a full in-depth one live so it's an experience that my group and I couldn't pass. I'm expecting it to be gruesome and shocking but also extremely informative.

The first time I saw a corpse was a few weeks ago and since then I have seen a few more. Despite this it is still weird seeing a soulless shell before you and so it is very intense to say the least. It is a great privilege to be exposed to this because so much of what we know about extending life arises critically from studying death during a very difficult time for people's loved ones.

The autopsy was of a male in their early 30s with a lot of injuries. The pathologist was meticulous in his process, observing all the tissues with the upmost care. Liver mortis was found (red-blue discolouration due to gravity) as well as rigor mortis (stiffness) and algor mortis (cooling). Unfortunately they also had a plethora of fractures and a lot of their organs were damaged.

Cause of death: Chest trauma and multiple organ rupture

One of the most gripping experiences I've ever had! Despite the potent aromas it was a good opportunity to visualise the organs in their true form. The gyri of the brain, the ruby red and sheen of the liver and the intricacy of the intact nerves and vessels. I cannot help but be amazed by the human body in all it's complexity.

Mind-blowing.

Because I know that this could be a very shocking experience for students I have decided to write some tips that I hope will be helpful.

- Keep hydrated and make sure to eat before you go especially if you're a squeamish person

- Expect strong foul smells so having a face mask helps

- Be careful where you step as sometimes you can find yourself in the splash zone

- Try to get lost in the physiology and pathology as it does help with an obviously sad stage of life

- Remember that nausea and anxiety are all human reactions and very normal responses. Don't feel bad and beat yourself up about it because there's nothing to be ashamed of. Get fresh air as soon as you feel you need it.

- If you feel any long term mental reactions do not hesitate to speak to someone for support as soon as you need it. Don't remain silent.

- As a medic just realise that you are there to learn and to apply your acquired knowledge in order to make your patient's lives better.

- Do something fun and decompress after as it can be an emotionally taxing experience

Some days I go into my lessons and find myself spending a few minutes of the day questioning why on earth I bothered to go in that day.

Studying has shown me that not everyone has the gift to teach and so sometimes you will find yourself regretting all your life choices.

Today was exactly that.

Absolutely painful to say the least.

I went in for a gastroenterology practical with not the best teacher in the world so I'm really going to end up teaching myself I suspect. Just lovely(!) Not to moan, but I do feel that if you do not like teaching please do your students a favour and don't go into it. *It's not by force.*

Can I get an Amen from my fellow uni students and graduates for this?!

26th March 2019

I am so drained so I think that this will probably be a short entry today.

I went to my Infectious Diseases practical at 10:15am. We discussed infectious and non-infectious rashes and also met a patient. She was a teenager presenting in an interesting way with chicken pox because children typically recover quickly. However, it turned out to be a blessing in disguise because her blood results were startling. Her haemoglobin, red blood cells and iron were severely low indicative of severe iron deficiency anaemia. During the consultation the patient complained of very heavy periods and so the ID professor referred her to the gynaecology department to get that sorted as this is the most likely cause of her severe anaemia.

Gastroenterology lecture.

Topic: Acute and chronic gastritis

One interesting thing I remember the lecturer saying was that some patients find that they feel less stomach complaints when they drink "heavy" liquor. He told us that this is because strong alcohol has been discovered to have necrolytic (numbing) effects whereas patients with these complaints tend to avoid wine which stimulates gastric secretions and so would make symptoms worse.

27th March 2019

Paediatrics practical.

Saw three patients today:
- A teenage girl with Crohn's disease (inflammatory disease of the bowels)

- Seven year old boy with post streptococcal glomerulonephritis (inflammation of the kidneys due to a previous bacterial infection)

- 10 year old boy with Henoch–Schönlein purpura (I hope you remember this disorder from a previous entry)

29th March 2019

Forensic Pathology practical.

Today's autopsy was one I will never forget-multiple fatalities due to carbon monoxide poisoning and house fire. The tissues were charred. The bones were disintegrated to dust, blackened and flaky. The internal organs were relatively intact apart from the brain which appeared like scrambled eggs (hopefully you're not eating breakfast). All the organs were red due to carbon monoxide gas because it forms an extremely strong bond with haemoglobin which intensifies the red colour.

Side note: That's why carbon monoxide alarms are very important so if you haven't already please get one ASAP!

Paediatrics practical.

Topic: Gastrointestinal disorders

Forensic Pathology lecture.

Topic: Stab wounds

We also went through some more neurology cases and as always I ended up writing some more helpful info:

Botulinum toxin A- can treat spasticity (stiffness)

The toxin Tetanospasmin mimics Upper Motor Neuron lesions

Damage above the sacrum > contracted bladder

Damage below the sacrum > atonic bladder

Three things I learnt today:

1. Congenital adrenal hyperplasia (CAH) leads to an increase in potassium and a decrease in sodium and chlorine

2. Haemolytic Urea Syndrome (HUS) is the most common cause of acute renal failure in babies

3. Hypervitaminosis (high storage of vitamins) can mimic UTI symptoms except that the urine is sterile

2nd April 2019

I had a bit of a lie in today but it literally felt like I had only had an hour's sleep.

Epidemiology practical @10:15am.

We did a review test that had 10 MCQs and thankfully that went well after which the professor covered exanthemous infections (i.e. infections associated with a rash such as chicken pox, rubella etc).

It was a very interesting lesson!

> The key thing I took from it was that you can give a vaccine to someone who has been exposed to chicken pox but only if it is less than 72 hours since the exposure.

Bought some McDonalds for lunch-got a cheeseburger and 2 large fries (the usual).

Gastroenterology lecture.

Three things I learnt today:

1. It is not advisable to give the antibiotic Clarithromycin for Helicobacter pylori infection treatment in areas where resistance to this antibiotic exceeds 15%. Surprisingly most of Europe exceeds this range so Amoxicillin would be more preferable in these circumstances.

2. Zollinger-Ellison syndrome is a tumour that produces lots of gastrin and is often located in the pancreas/duodenum. If you have a patient with multiple ulcers this should be ruled out as a differential diagnosis.

3. DO NOT give barium to patients where perforation or penetration of ulcers is suspected because this can increase the risk of chemical peritonitis (injury that

occurs when chemicals leak into the abdominal cavity).

3rd April 2019

General medicine practical.
CANCELLED!
(Yes! Lie in it is. Yay!)

Psychiatry practical.

We conversed with a female patient with post traumatic stress disorder and another female patient who lost her son and developed psychosis with auditory hallucinations.

Epidemiology lecture.

Topic: Food-borne diseases including Shigella, Salmonella and Typhoid fever

Side note: I cannot understand how people have been raised at home. It is a shock to realise how many do not have sufficient home training at all. Apparently only 66% of women and 34% of men wash their hands after using the loo. The mind boggles. Please guys for all that is good in the world make sure you wash your hands! JHEEZE!

(THANK GOD FOR ANTIBAC!)

Parasitology lecture.

Topic: Worm infections including Neurocysticercosis, Toxocariasis, Trichuriasis and Echinococcosis

(I know a mouthful, right?)

I leave it to you to research them for homework tonight, okay?

Clue: You won't find these in a Harry Potter book mate even though they sound like they really should be.

The lecturer even gave us an insight into what it was like working abroad in Libya, Angola and Vietnam. He's so passionate about his field. One day that will be me.

Tropical medicine is clearly where my passion lies considering the amount of times I bang on about it.

4th April 2019

Paediatrics practical.

Patient 1: Seven year old with exudate in the oral cavity, ecchymosis (bruises) and petechiae (pin-point spots)

Dx= Infectious mononucleosis caused by the Epstein Barr Virus (EBV)

Patient 2: Three year old that was very irritable, fatigued and displayed Opsoclonus myoclonus (also called dancing eye syndrome which is a neurological condition normally associated with neuroblastoma)

Surprisingly the abdominal ultrasound was negative for neuroblastoma.

Dx= To be confirmed with further investigation

10th April 2019

General medicine practical.

We went to the simulation centre which was quite fun as we were learning how to deliver babies. I delivered my first baby today (I know it's only a doll but let me have this moment)! The teacher even added fake lubricant to show how slippery this process is. Thankfully all of us managed to safely deliver the gooey baby without it shooting straight out of our hands so hopefully the same can be said if we end up having to do the real thing.

*fingers crossed

Tip 1: Maintain a tight but safe grip because they'll literally feel like jelly

Tip 2: Simulations are obviously easier so expect a lot of screams, the smell of blood and possibly faeces in real life

Psychiatry practical.

It was arranged to be a review lesson but it ended up being a random discussion about society and how corruption is in every nation in some shape or form. I can't help but admire a medic that thinks outside the box because they are few and far between. We even discussed that when we think about medicine we have to ask ourselves about what we actually cure instead of just treat. We really need to put more effort into preventative medicine.

I know. Completely off topic but it does make you think. It was a very deep discussion to be fair.

Infectious diseases lecture.

Topic: HIV/AIDS
(I would really like to give my thoughts on it's origin but for the sake of peace I will leave that for another time).

Parasitology lecture.

Schistosomiasis (infection due to flatworms called schistosomes)

GOOGLE ALERT!

General medicine lecture.

Topic: Geriatrics and gerontology (ageing)

I have a soft spot for the elderly so this was the first general medicine lecture I actually enjoyed. (Sorry to my GPs if you are offended LOL).

> Quote of the day: "And in the end, it's not the years in your life that count. It's the life in your years."

*mic drop

PURE FACTS!

11th April 2019

Looks like the sore throat's here to stay. (Guess that's what I get for not getting honey and lemon again. Us medics are the epitome of do as I say but not as I do).

I really struggled to get ready at 9:20am for my paediatrics practical. I cannot wait to come home to rest because I am so knackered. I will try my upmost best to not doze off during the lesson but I can't make any promises.

And I don't think the weather forecast helps to be fair.

Afternoon rain and 65% humidity. Fantastic (!)

It's as if I'm still in the UK.

Paediatrics practical.

Unfortunately we saw a 5 months old girl with severe malnutrition and rickets. It was sad because unfortunately her mother wasn't feeding her appropriately so she only weighed about 3kg which is the birth of a newborn. The mother has not returned since her admission so hopefully she'll be adopted into a good family soon. Things like this really highlight how blessed I am. Sometimes you need to appreciate what you have because there is always someone worse off than you.

Tongue fasciculations (muscle twitches)
Floppy baby syndrome (lack of muscle tone, muscle weakness, and lack of muscle control)
Hyporeflexia (low reflex responses)
Hypotonia (low muscle tone)

DDx= Spinal muscular dystrophy (rare disorder that results in loss of motor neurons and muscle wasting)

Sadly if this is the case the prognosis is poor but the doctors are trialling a new drug on the market called SPINRAZA which may extend her lifespan.

We also saw a young boy diagnosed with lymphoma and he is currently on chemotherapy which has probably led to his present fungal infection due to *Trichosporum*. His X-ray results were shocking as they revealed severe inflammation of the lungs which have not responded well to multiple antifungals so unfortunately it isn't looking good. The poor boy has had to go on life support so I can only imagine how his parents are dealing with this.

Medicine is not easy. At all.

Forensic Pathology practical.

We saw multiple examples of firearms and different types of wounds. Ballistics is actually quite intriguing.

Tip 1: Entry wounds can be classified into contact, close, near range and distant range depending on how close the firearm is to the victim.

Tip 2: Wounds = entry + exit + wound tract

Tip 3: Guns have a grip, trigger, hammer with a pin, barrel and muzzle.

12th April 2019

Happy birthday sis!
Time flies.

Paediatrics practical.

We met a teenage male patient who was diagnosed with Type 1 Diabetes about a decade ago. He was coming in for his yearly check up. He had been prescribed insulin Novorapid (short acting form) to be taken three times a day and Levenir (long acting form) to take in the evening before bed time. Quite smart actually because the short acting form will help stabilise his glucose after he eats his meals and the one at night will gradually stabilise his glucose whilst he sleeps. He has been advised to have six small meals a day (3 meals and 3 snacks). He has also been made aware of bread units (~12g of carbs) which would help him to better regulate his carbohydrate intake.

The professor also explained to us why the risk of Diabetes is more pronounced during pregnancy and this is because sex hormones have anti-insulin effects (i.e. they work against insulin). Also the fastest acting hormone is adrenaline which is why diabetic patients get pale, sweaty and develop tachycardia etc.

So the teacher urged us to be able to decipher the differences between how diabetic ketoacidosis vs hyperglycaemia presents because medical students tend to get them confused:

Diabetic ketoacidosis	Hyperglycaemia
(A serious problem that can happen in people with diabetes if their body starts to run out of insulin)	(Elevated blood glucose)
Reddish cheeks Reduced eye pressure Dry skin and mucous membranes Dehydration Reduced skin elasticity Difficult to feel pulse Reduced tendon reflexes	Pale Normal eye pressure Increased tendon reflexes Babinski sign

Parasitology practical.

(My fav! As you should know by now :-p)

Topic: *Taenia solium* (pork tapeworm), *Taenia saginata* (beef tapeworm) and *Hymenolepis nana (dwarf tapeworm)*

When you get a chance please get your hands on the book "*The Woman with a Worm in Her Head: And Other True Stories of Infectious Disease by Pamela Nagami*" and prepare to be amazed.

Forensic pathology lecture.

For the first time ever I have decided to bunk the lecture since my sore throat is giving me trouble. I'm actually supposed to be singing at a Christian union event tomorrow so I do hope that I'll be better before then. #altos

5th May 2019

I ended up bunking the paediatrics practical because I had a sore throat (again).

Parasitology practical.

Topic: Chagas disease/American Trypanosomiasis (caused by the parasite Trypanosoma carried by the tsetse fly)

No matter how many times I see the word tsetse I cannot seem to pronounce it correctly.

ME: Hey Google? How do you pronounce the word tsetse."

Google: SEET-see, TSEET-see or TSET-sə

Oh great that helps (!)
Now I'm confused again.

8th May 2019

Gastroenterology practical.

CANCELLED.

Thank God for that.

Fast forward to the end of June…

Days, weeks and months have passed by because it is now exam time so I haven't had time to write any entries I'm afraid.

29th June 2019

I am well into exam season and have successfully completed five exams with just three more to go.

I have officially reached a plateau. I was so pumped to revise for the previous exams pushing myself and maintaining my revision targets and now burnout has set it.

My body is drained. My mind is bombarded with information. I'm constantly dozing off and waking up early for revision is extremely taxing now. I have headaches and have found myself re-reading the same sentences over and over again.

My mum said that I should take a break but as a medic it's so difficult to do so because it doesn't seem like there is time to fit it in. There is so much revision to get through and so little time.

The next exam is Psychiatry which highlights the importance of looking after your mental health and psychological support yet during exam season my colleagues and I find ourselves in desperate need of this very thing. How ironic?

Medicine is what I love but like a marriage it's something that you constantly have to work at. Some days you find yourself in awe lost in the pages of your cardiology textbook oozing with excitement. Whilst on other days you sit fixated on the wall contemplating your regrets and the decisions that got you to this very point. However, in writing out my thoughts it is as if I have gradually distressed my mind.

It has just hit me that burnout is not only normal but inevitable. I spent many years aiming for medical school with full knowledge that this will happen. Sometimes you have to be honest with yourself. Was this a decision that was forced upon me or did I go into medicine on my own accord? Since it was my decision (thanks to the support of my family) I really have to remember that sometimes you really have to push through. Medicine is not for everyone and you cannot go into it expecting unicorns and rainbows.

You will cry sometimes.

You will be moody sometimes.

You will constantly find yourself nearing close to hypoglycaemia because you missed a meal again.

You will want to scream.

You will want to give in.

But…

If there's one bit of advice you take from this journal it would be.

DON'T.

You are not alone.

It might be hard to express your vulnerability but find someone you can talk to with swift urgency. Too many medics have lost their mental stability because of how rigorous this career is and I don't want you to be another. Speak to your family or a friend that understands. It may also help to speak to the doctors at your university because they have gone through the exact same thing.

Have a break!
Go for a walk!
Meditate and pray!

Write out your frustrations in your own journal because trust me it is therapeutic.

Write out your worries on a piece of paper then tear them up and dispose of them.

In essence you are predicting your victory.

You will beat this but the change begins today. You have to put your self-care first or all your dreams will be put under jeopardy.

Why you ask?

Because you owe it to yourself.

You owe it to the future you safely delivering you first baby, pure elation evident on the mother's eyes.

You owe it to the 70 year old battling with stage 4 cancer as you help make such a difficult time slightly more bearable.

And you owe it to the medical student sheepishly walking into your practice shaking with anxiety. You will be there to say that you were once in their shoes and therefore can give them encouragement based on your experience which helps them to push through.

When my Mum said I should take a break in all it's simplicity I have come to the realisation that she was in fact right.

Summer exam results:

18/05/2019

Clinical Oncology
Passed with flying colours

03/06/2019

Paediatrics
Passed with flying colours

08/06/2019

Forensic Pathology
Passed with flying colours

10/06/2019

Infectious diseases, Epidemiology &
Parasitology
Passed with flying colours

21/06/2019

Internal Medicine
Passed with flying colours

08/07/2019

Obstetrics and Gynaecology

> Passed with flying colours
>
> 15/08/2019
>
> General Medicine
> Passed (just about lol)
>
> SUCCESS!!!

Three things I have learnt this year:

1. I really REALLY do love Tropical medicine as a specialty

2. When you have a good support network around you the impossible can become possible

3. I'm always hungry LOL

Until next time…

Acknowledgements

Firstly I must give honour to my Lord and Saviour Jesus Christ who has open doors for me in rooms I had no knowledge of. I am thankful for his favour and so I have to give all glory to him.

Thanks to the inspiring physicians that taught me throughout my medical school career. This includes Professor Radka Komitova, Professor Vanya Rangelova, Professor Galia Popova-Daskalova, Professor Julia Nikolova, Professor Oliana Boykinova, Professor Yana Merdzhanova, Professor Mariya Spasova, Professor Ivan Tsranchev, Professor Pavel Timonov, Professor Krasimir Kraev and Professor Dimitar Vuchev to name but a few.

I would also like to thank my best friend of 16 plus years and fellow physician for taking the plunge with me as we pursued medicine together abroad and for being there as a support and encouragement in the good times and bad. Medical school would not have been the same without you so for this I am extremely thankful.

In closing, I must give my gratitude to my family.

For instilling within us the yearning to read things for ourselves, critically analyse and learn more each day.

For the long nights helping me with my school work when I just couldn't seem to get it.

For your wisdom and advice during the many times I was close to throwing in the towel.

For encouraging me to follow my dreams.

For the prayers for my mental strength and my safekeeping.

For funding my studies and sending me some of my favourite snacks across the waters.

For being my greatest cheerleaders.

For trying your best to make revision at home manageable during the Christmas season when January exams were close.

For taking me to and from the airport so much we know the route by heart now.

For encouraging me to write this book in the first place.

For my younger sister pointing me in the right direction on that train ride to Central London that got me inspired to put this together.

For my younger brother reading my rough draft and for letting me know the new things he learnt by reading it.

Dear family.
I am because of you.
I will because of you.

Xx Thank you to my Grandparents, Mum, Dad, brother and sister (and of course my cat Liquorice lol).

And this is also inspired by the loved ones that have shaped me into who I am today but have gone on. I will not forget you.

Grandad M
Grandad J
Mother M
Great Grandad M
My Godmother L

www.ingramcontent.com/pod-product-compliance
Lightning Source LLC
Chambersburg PA
CBHW070417220526
45466CB00004B/1436